HOUSE OF WELLNESS INSTANT HOME REMEDIES

Every chapter has been crafted by my passion for holistic wellbeing and belief that true health is amalgamation of mind, body and spirit.

Happy reading !!!

Dr. Khushbu Mehta

Disclaimer

While every effort has been made to verify the authenticity of the information contained in the book, remedies prescribed in the book are not intended as a substitute for medical consultation with a physician. The publisher and the author are in no way liable for the use of the information contained in the book.

Pregnant women, small children, and aged weak people cannot take any therapies mentioned in the book without consulting your physician and supervision.

Additionally, it is essential to recognize that individual health conditions and sensitivities can vary greatly, and what may be suitable for one person might not be appropriate for another. Therefore, readers are strongly advised to exercise caution and seek professional medical advice before embarking on any therapies or treatments suggested in this book. It is always best to prioritize your health and well-being by consulting a qualified healthcare provider who can offer personalized guidance based on your specific needs and circumstances. Remember, your health should always come first, and this book should be seen as a source of information to complement, not replace, professional medical advice and care.

Contents

About The Author

"If you want to shine like a sun, first burn like a sun."

She strongly believes in this quote as it firmly relates to her journey. She is Dr. Khushbu Mehta, a physiotherapist, a clinical nutritionist and a Bioresonance program handler.

Her passion for allied therapies developed since childhood. Her grandfather wished for her to heal people without medications and god gifted her with this beautiful healing profession of physiotherapy.

In her initial years of studying Physiotherapy, she used to visit various charitable trusts for internships and even assisted her aunt (Dr. Dwarika) and uncle (Dr. Nitin) for various surgeries.

She passed out physiotherapy in 2010 with internship in Wockhardt hospital (Fortis, Mumbai). For over 2 years, she solely practiced as a physiotherapist in a local charitable institute and got people heal. Along with practising physiotherapy, she also did various courses on advanced physiotherapy like dry needling, cupping, taping, Mulligan, acupressure and acupuncture therapies.

During her pregnancy in 2012, she studied clinical nutrition program and then started to cure patients with two magic hands - physiotherapy and nutrition. She got miraculous results with the combination of both the therapies and patient started getting cured in shorter span of time.

Now with passing time of practicing physiotherapy for 13 years and clinical nutrition for 11 years and her love for other allied therapies, she is now the Head of Department of GKM Medical and Wellness centre. She is following her passion and providing selfless service at the centre and curing people using various allied therapies. Recently, she has stepped into the world of research and have submitted research articles in 'Indian Association of Scientific Research' in 2023.

Achievments Of author:

- Kapol Samaj Gaurav award (March 2022)

- Ghatkopar Gaurav award (June 2022)

- Bharat Gaurav Puraskar (February 2023)

- Best Physiotherapy award (May 2023)

- Best Achiever's award (Magic Book of Record, July 2023)

- Best Iconic Doctor of the year 2023 (India's Top 50 Legendary Women's Award 2023)

- Prerna Star Award 2023 -Achievers book of records

- Bharat Gaurav Ratna Shri Samman Council - 2023

- Cerificate of appreciation from Indian women history museum 2023

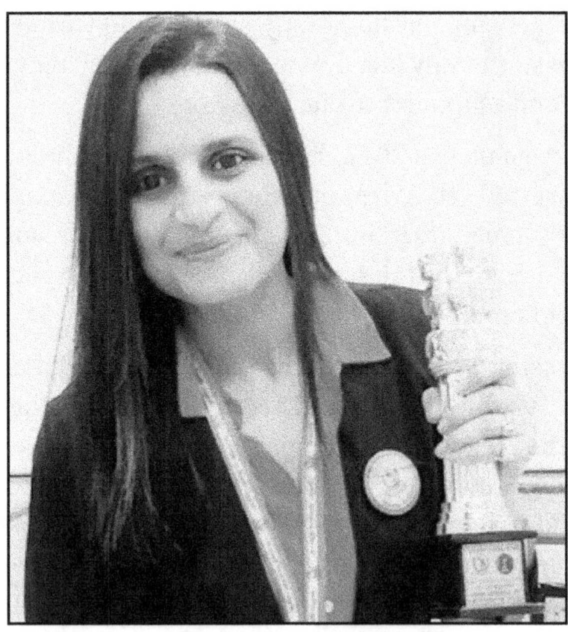

Dr. Khushbu Mehta

Acknowledgements

All my dreams of serving society have come true and all the I have got the appreciation for the same only with the teachings and blessings of my parents

Mr. Deepak Mehta & Mr. Chandresh Mehta,

Mrs. Nimisha Mehta & Mrs. Bhavna Mehta

Trust, love and support of my husband Mr. Jenil Mehta and

My daughter Ms. Vrriyaa Mehta

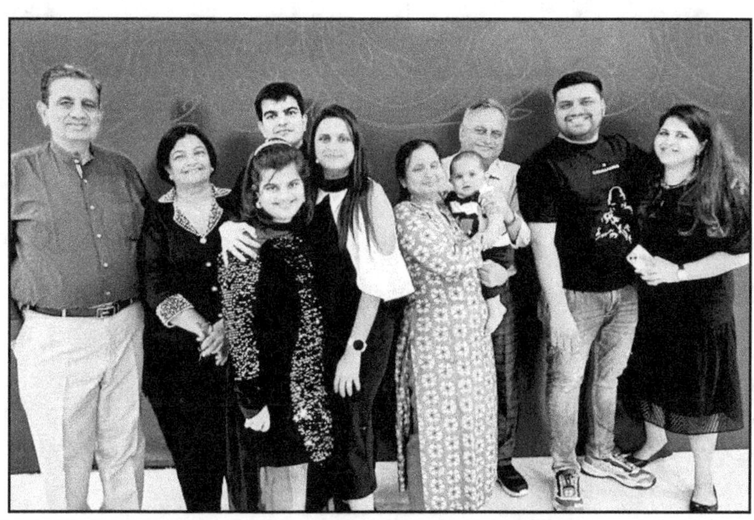

I dedicate all my awards, achievements and appreciation to my beloved family.

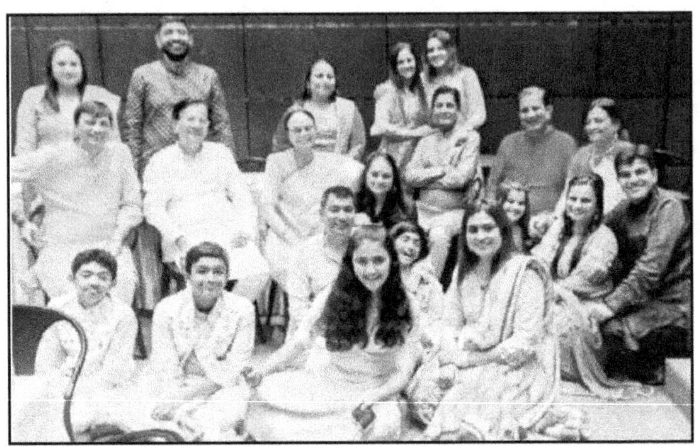

This book is dedicated in loving memory of

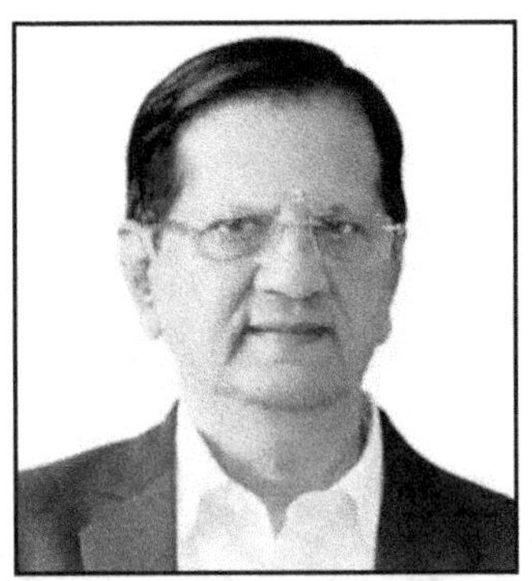

Mr. Navinchandra Mehta

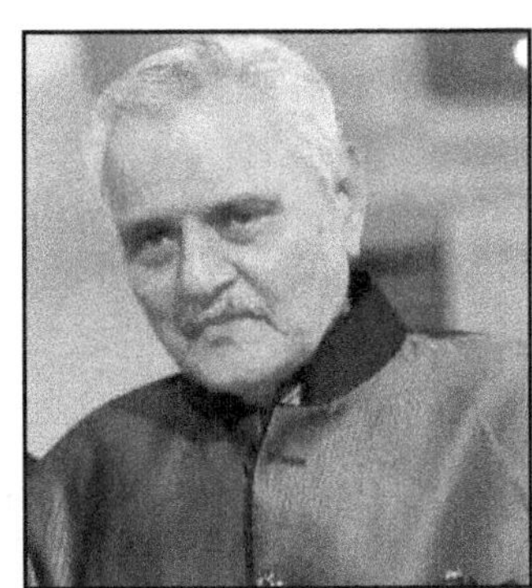

Mr. Rameshchandra Mehta

Thank you to all my co-authors for spreading the knowledge to society through this book:

- **Dr. Foram Shah**   - **Dt. Gargi P. Shah**

- **Dt. Nidhi Parekh**   - **Rap. Kinjal Patel**

About Co- Authors

Dr. Foram Shah - Physiotherapist - 10 years of experience - currently working in Shree Ghatkopar Kapol Mahajan Medical & Wellness Centre as head of physiotherapy department - Aim is to provide best healthcare services through physiotherapy to make lives pain-free and restriction free.

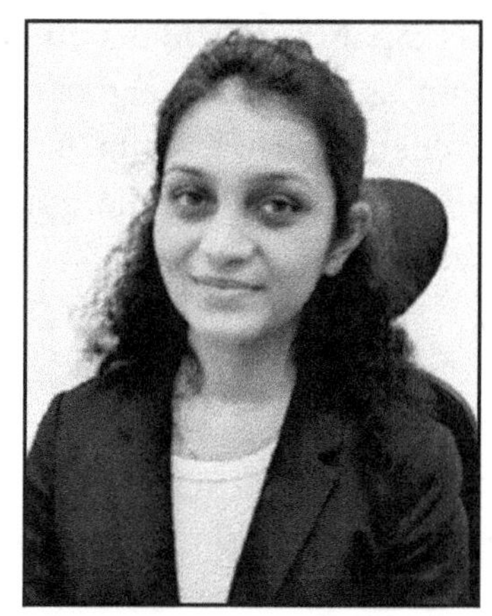

Dt. Gargi Shah - Masters in Specialised Dietetics (Specialisation in Diabetes & Cardiac Nutrition) - 1 year of experience in Shree Ghatkopar Kapol Mahajan Medical & Wellness Centre as clinical nutritionist - aim is to prevent and reverse diseases through optimum nutrition

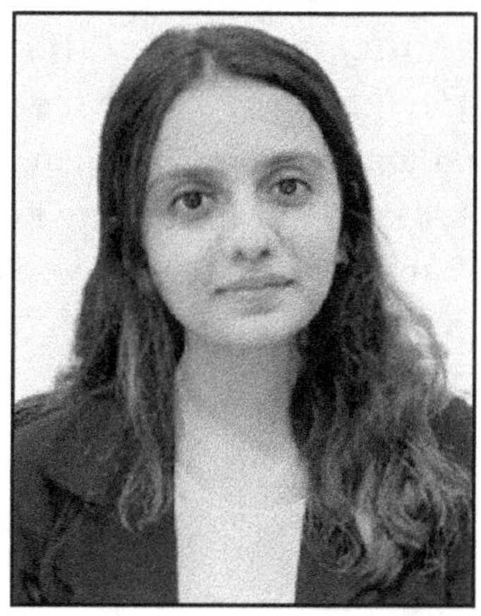

Rap. Kinjal Patel - Acupuncture and acupressure specialist - work experience of 2 years in Shree Ghatkopar Kapol Mahajan Medical & Wellness Centre as head of department in allied therapy - aim is to provide wellness with allied therapies without any side effects

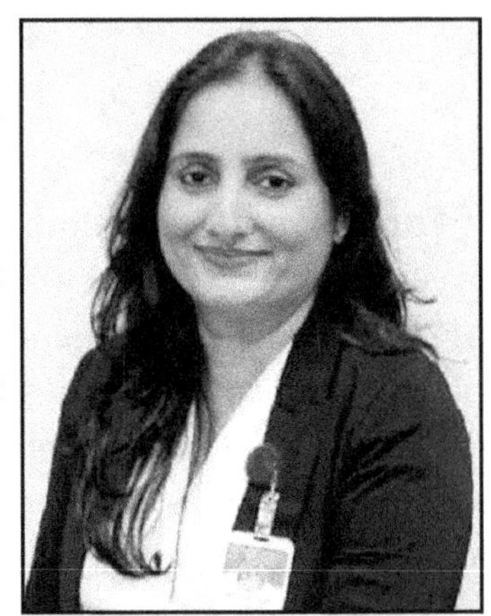

Mrs. Nidhi Parekh - Weight management specialist - work experience of 2 years in Shree Ghatkopar Kapol Mahajan Medical & Wellness Centre - helping people to be fit and healthy with best of her knowledge

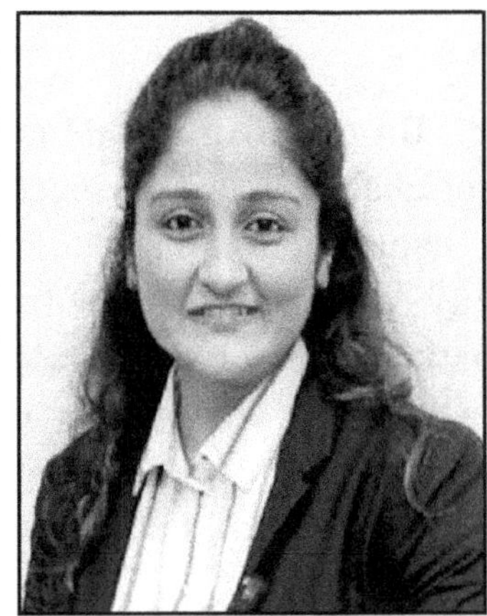

Heartily Thanks to Shree Ghatkopar Kapol Mahajan Wellness and Medical Centre

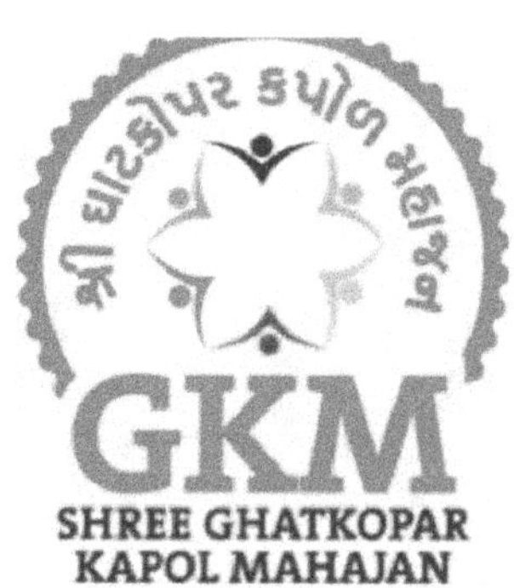

For giving me this opportunity of serving societywith help of new technologies and our Indian ancient methods. This centre taught me to take Indian culture and new technology together to cure patients and this innovative way of curing people and inspired us to step in the world of research and write various research articles and case studies in Indian association of scientific research journal.

Heartfelt thanks for putting faith in us and always encouraging us to pursue our dreams.

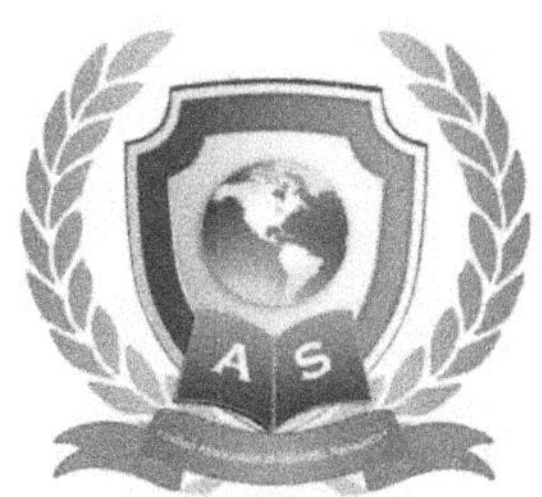

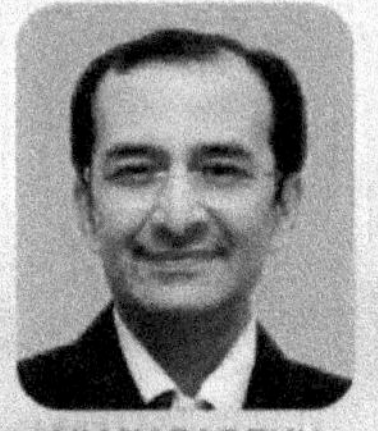
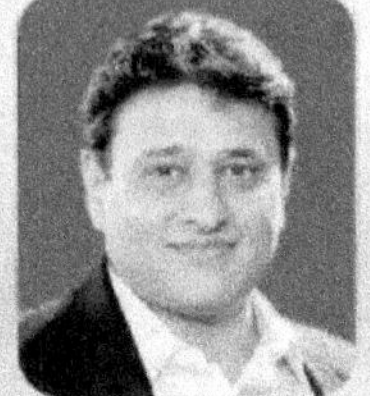
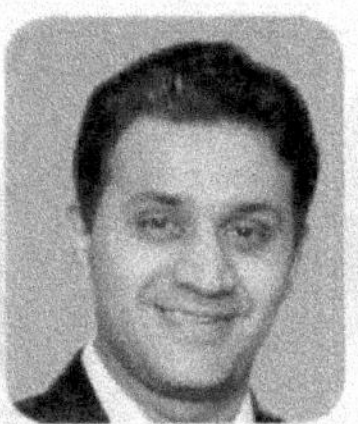
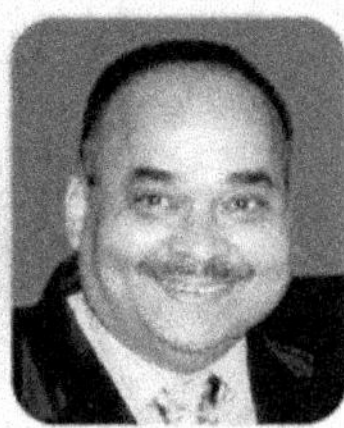
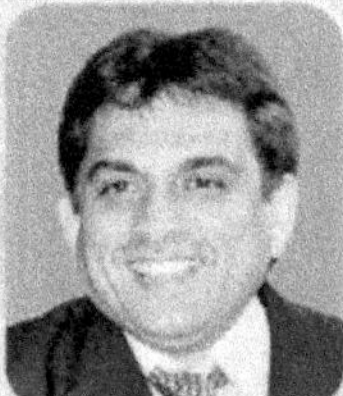
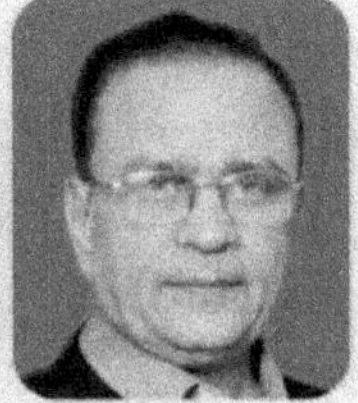
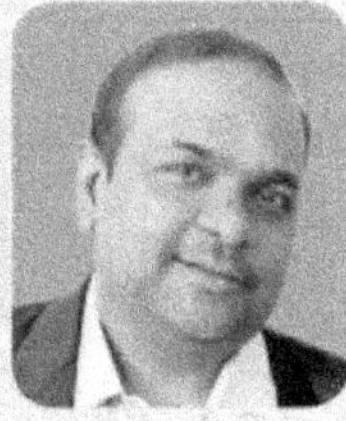
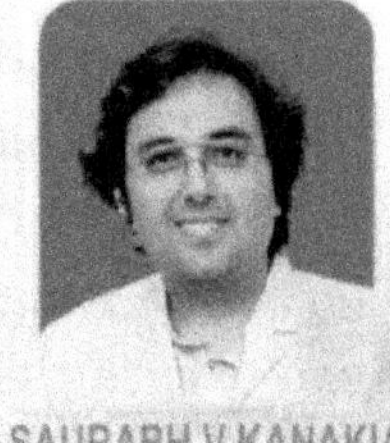

Thanks to president of the centre Mr. Vijay Parekh, and vice president Mr. Prashant Parekh

And all the committee members Mr. Hitesh Mehta, Vipul Mehta, Mr. Rajesh Parekh, Mr. Saurabh Kanakia, Mr. Bharat Muni, Mr. Vinay Vora for giving me opportunity to head the wellness department and provide best of services to all communities.

About the Book

The book you hold in your hands is a comprehensive guide to instant remedies, drawing upon a rich tapestry of traditional and modern healing practices. In its pages, you will find a treasure trove of knowledge encompassing Dadi ma ke Gharelu Nuskhe (the age-old home remedies passed down through generations), Kadha (herbal concoctions), specific foods for healing, Acupressure points, and Mudras (hand gestures) carefully curated to address five common conditions that affect us in our daily lives.

This book aims to empower you with the tools to take control of your health and well-being, offering accessible solutions that can be easily incorporated into your daily routine. Whether you are seeking relief from common ailments like headaches, digestive issues, stress, insomnia, or muscle pain, you will discover practical and effective remedies that can provide relief without the need for complex medical interventions.

With a blend of age-old wisdom and modern insights, this book is a valuable resource for those seeking natural and holistic approaches to health. It is a testament to the power of simple, yet effective remedies that have been passed down through generations and adapted to fit our contemporary lifestyles. Dive in, explore, and embark on a journey towards better health through the wisdom contained within these pages.

Introduction

In today's fast-paced world, where desk jobs, junk food, stress, anxiety, and environmental changes have become common trends, our health is facing numerous challenges. A sedentary lifestyle has led to a rise in obesity rates and an increase in health issues that affect people of all age groups. Many individuals find themselves struggling with gastric issues, knee pain, and other common ailments that impact their daily lives.

In the midst of these health challenges, there is a growing awareness of the need for sustainable solutions that address the root causes of these problems. People are seeking effective remedies that not only provide relief but also promote long-term well-being. This is where our book comes in.

Our book caters to individuals of all ages and backgrounds, recognizing that health is a universal concern. Whether you are a young professional struggling with the effects of a sedentary lifestyle or a middle-aged individual battling obesity, this book is here to support you on your journey to better health.

We understand that it can be overwhelming to navigate the sea of information available on health and wellness. That's why we have compiled the most relevant and effective strategies in one comprehensive resource. By drawing from the wisdom of Vedic health culture, we offer time-tested practices and remedies that have been passed down through generations.

By embracing the principles and practices outlined in this book, you will discover how to keep your organs happy and fit, how to find relief from common ailments, and how to approach wellness. We believe that true wellness is not just the absence of disease but a state of complete well-being that encompasses the physical, mental, emotional, and spiritual aspects of our lives.

We invite you to embark on a transformative journey towards holistic wellness. Let the House of Wellness be your guide as you navigate the challenges of modern life and reclaim your health. Together, let us discover the sustainable solutions that will help you thrive and live a fulfilling life with holistic approach.

Chapter 1: Instant Remedies for Cough

1. Add 1/4th teaspoon of ginger juice with 1 teaspoon of honey.

2. Try sipping warm turmeric milk before you sleep - 1/2 teaspoon turmeric with one cup milk. Add a dash of black pepper and some honey.

3. Having 2-3 dates with 5 sips of warm water everyday also helps thinning of cough.

4. Having Roasted chana 6-7 pieces before sleep with warm water also helps for cough removal.

5. 1 cup of warm water with 1/2 teaspoon turmeric powder, 1 pinch salt and 1/2 spoon dry ginger (saunth) powder thrice a day.

6. Boil cabbage leaves in water and take steam with this water for 10 minutes at least twice a day.

7. You can also keep cabbage leaves near your chest at night to remove cough.

8. Keep sipping on hot fluids throughout the day to melt away the cough.

9. Eat a slice of pineapple or drink 100 ml (1/2 cup) of fresh pineapple juice three times a day.

10. A salt and water gargle may help soothe a scratchy throat and break up mucus that causes you to cough. Mixing 1/4 to 1/2 teaspoon of salt with 1 cup of warm water can help to relieve irritation.

11.   Active cycle of breathing technique: this combines different breathing techniques that helps to clear mucus from the lungs.

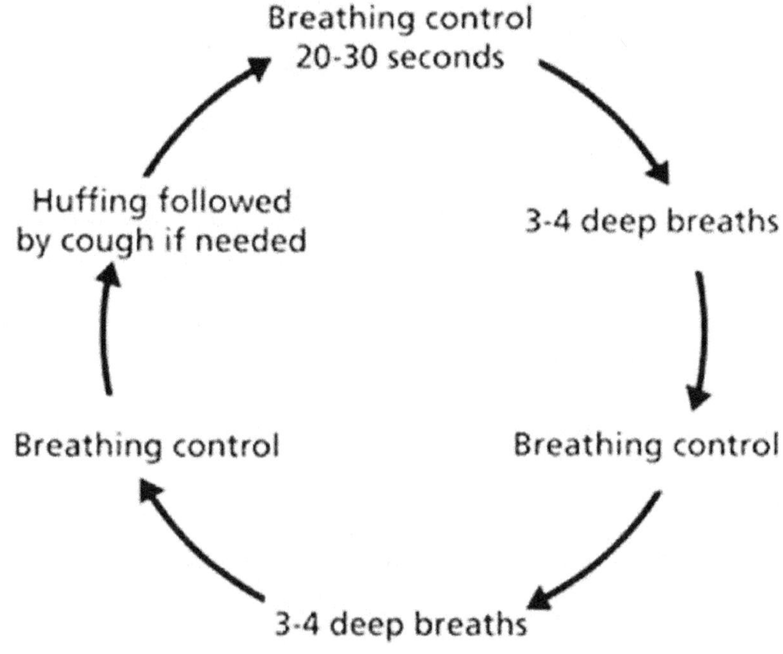

Active Cycle of Breathing Technique

12.   2- 3 Tulsi leaves on empty stomach or boil tulsi leaves 6-7 leaves in water and drink the water.

13.   Give pressure for 1 minute for 5-7 times in a day

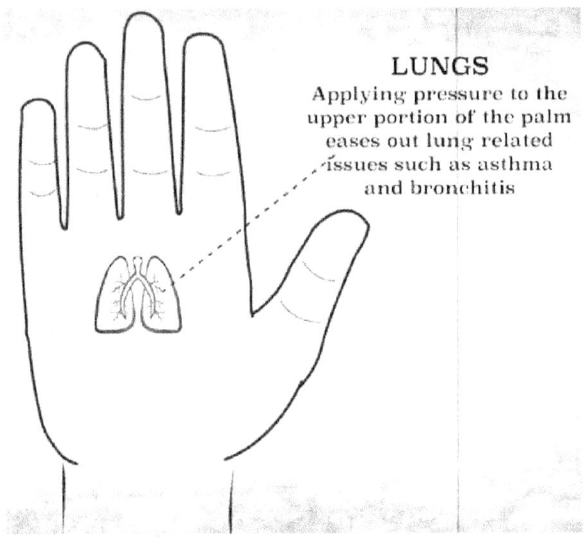

14.   Press this point 5-7 times in a day

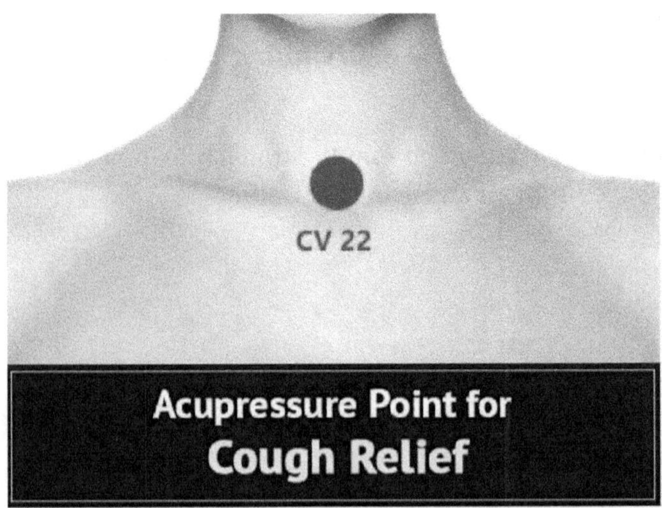

15.   Do this mudra whenever you are free

- Removes speech defects
- Relieves asthma
- Tones up the throat, airways and the lungs
- Helps to calm your mind
- Cures thyroid problems
- Cures skin diseases

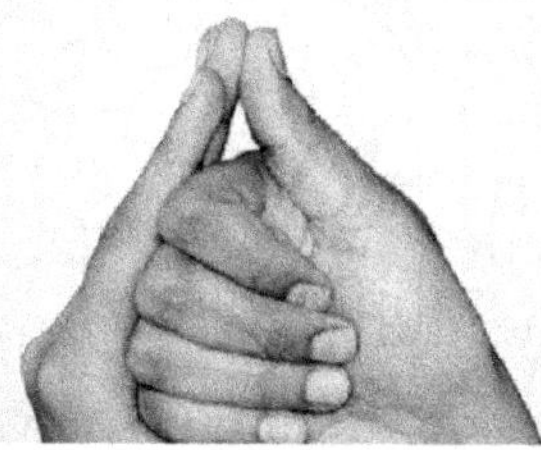

- Cures cough generated problems like asthma, pneumonia, tuberculosis.
- Generates heat in body which helps in problems of colds, catarrh and coughs.
- Removes the excess fat from body.

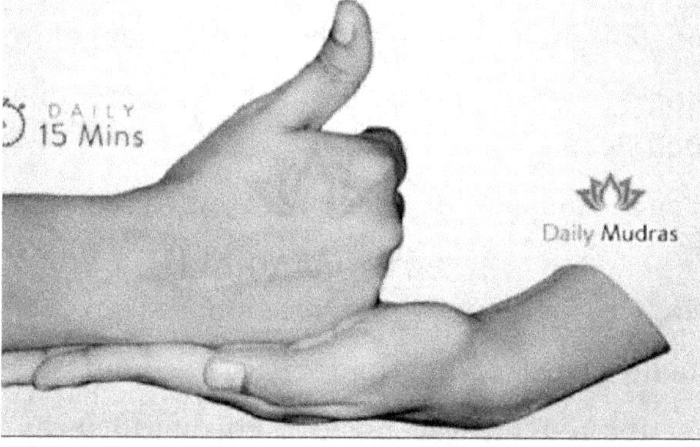

MUDRAS FOR YOUR THROAT PROBLEMS

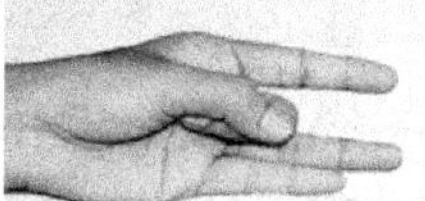
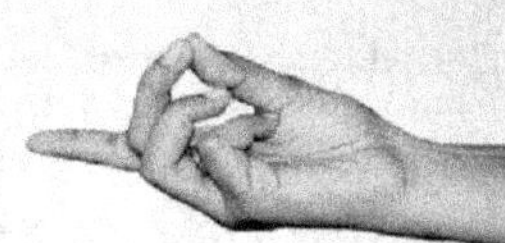

SHUNYA MUDRA

BRONCHIAL MUDRA

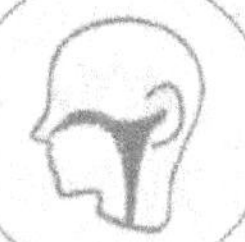

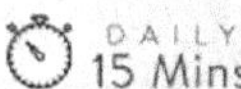

Chapter 2: Remedies for Insomnia (No sleep)

1. Wash your hands and legs with cold water and apply some ghee on your forehead for good sleep.

2. Have 1/4 th teaspoon of nutmeg powder (Jaiphal) and 1/2 teaspoon turmeric powder with 1 cup of warm milk at night also induces sleep.

3. Piparmul powder (long pepper root) also helps for good sleep.

4. Applying cow`s ghee on feet before sleep.

5. Having 2-3 grams of poppy seeds with honey before bedtime.

6. Having cold mixture of fennel seeds + sugar + milk also helps in good sleep.

7. Having 1 teaspoon of honey before bed also induces faster sleep.

8. Having rice for dinner also induces good sleep.

9. Eat lighter meals at night and at least two hours before bed.

10. Repeating a mantra or positive affirmations repeatedly can help focus and calm your mind and help in sleep.

11. Aroma therapy with lavender oil at bedtime helps to calm mind and induce sleep.

12. Nabhi Kriya, or oiling therapy, is a simple yet effective practice. Put 3 drops of lavender oil in your belly button, massage for 5 minutes before sleeping and keep it overnight. This aids in better sleep.

13. Stay active, but exercise earlier in the day.

14. Take a hot shower or bath at the end of your day.

15. Avoid screens one to two hours before bed.

16. Keep your bedroom dark and cool, and try to use it only for sleeping.

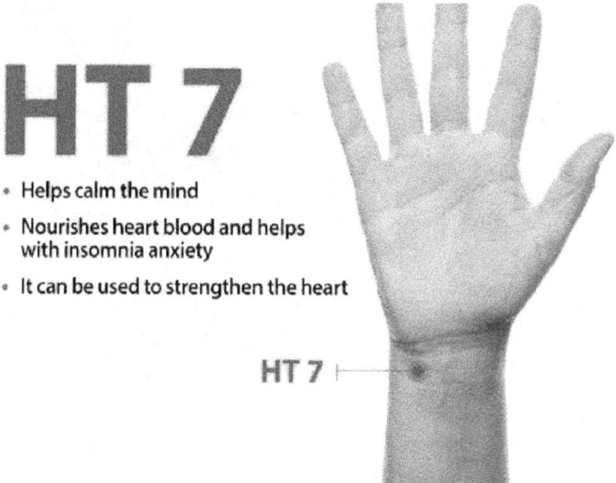

Chapter 3:
Instant Remedies
for Swelling

1. Crushing 5 to 6 cloves and applying its paste on the Swelling reduces the swelling.

2. Applying a paste of mustard and black salt relieves swelling.

3. Applying turmeric and lime reduces the swelling.

4. Applying turmeric and salt cures swelling caused by bruises or sprains.

5. Drinking radish leaf juice cures swelling.

6. Grinding tulsi leaves and applying them on the swelling reduces the swelling.

7. A easy self-care practise known as the RICE method helps to reduce swelling and promote healing.

- Rest the injured area

- Ice the injured area to reduce pain, swelling/inflammation

- Compression: wrap the area to reduce swelling

- Elevate the body part above the heart when resting to reduce swelling

RICE Method

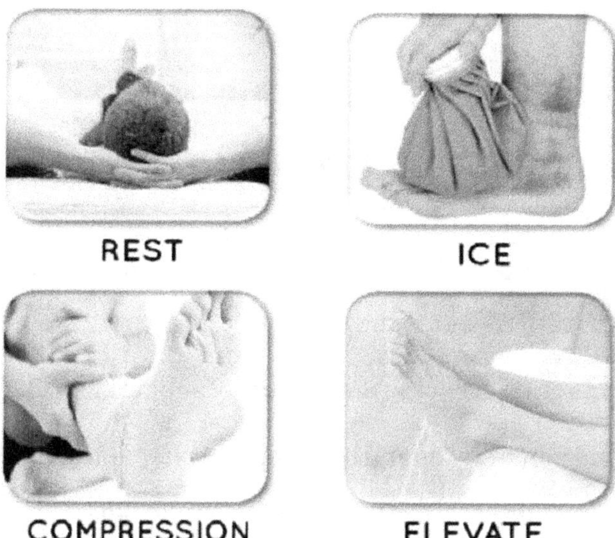

8.   Massage this kidney point 5-7 times in a day for 1 minute
This will reduce swelling, Inflammation and urinary problems

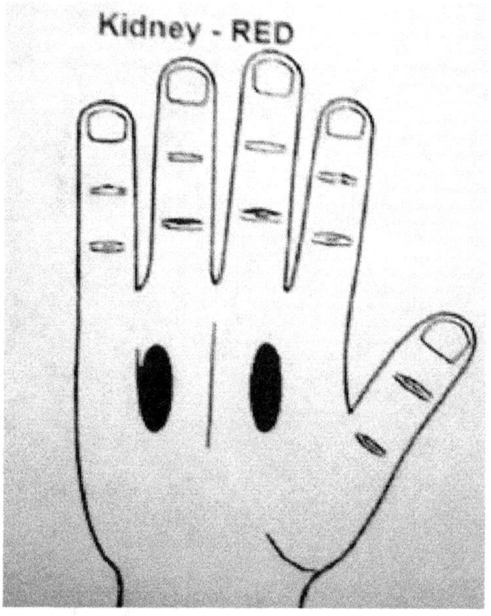

Chapter 4: Remedies for Ear pain/Tinnitus

1.   Heat clove of garlic in oil and putting a drop of that oil in the ear cures ear infections and ear Pain.

2.   Drops of Tulsi juice in the ear cures ear pain and itching.

3.   Grind fennel seeds and boil them in water and apply the steam on the painful ear to cure deafness and ringing in the ear.

4.   Drops of white onion juice in the ear twice a day cures ear ache.

      Gently massage this point 2-3 times in day for pain, infection, tinnitus

5.   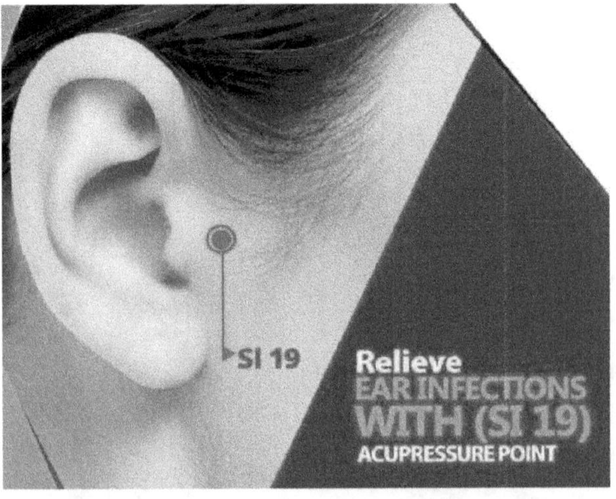

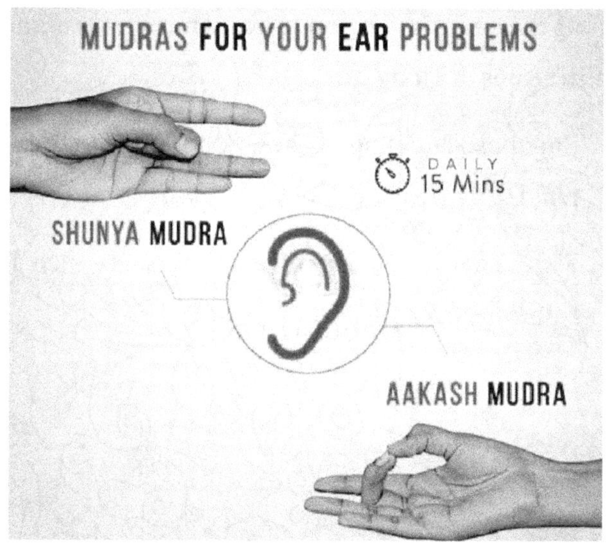

7.   Herbal moxa sticks

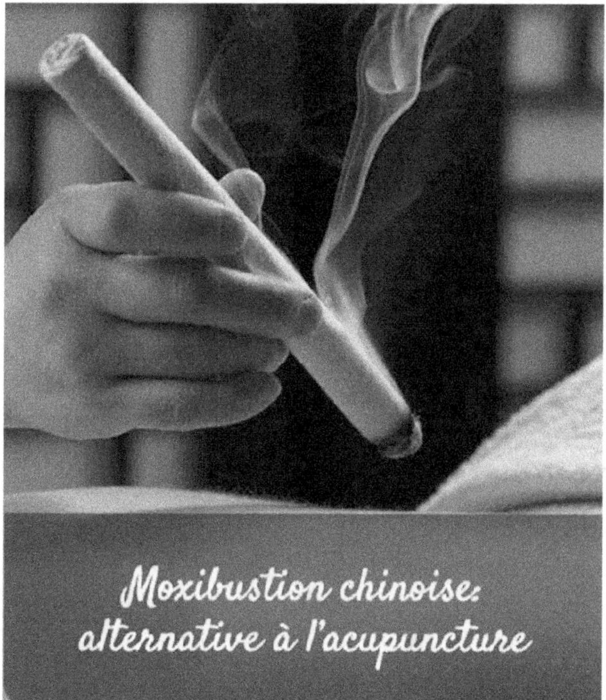

8.   Here is the best diet for you to avoid hearing loss and other ear health issues in a long run.

- Bananas: The magnesium-rich fruit is all that your ears needed as a regular diet.

- Fish: The Omega3 and Vitamin D are rich in fish like salmon and tuna.

- Dark Chocolate

- Oranges

- Milk Products

- Green Leaves

Chapter 5: Instant Remedies for Back Pain

1. Eating carrom and jaggery in equal measure in the morning and evening cures back pain.

2. Taking dry ginger powder with warm water cures back pain.

3. Boiling five dates and adding half a teaspoon of fenugreek to it and drinking it cures back pain.

4. Heat dry ginger powder and asafoetida in a oil and massage with it relieves back pain or body stiffness. Joint pain is also cured.

5. Dry ginger powder, garlic and carrom seeds heat it in mustard oil and massage which helps to relieve in back pain and joint aches.

6. Spinach, broccoli, sweet potatoes, berries, watermelon, green tea, beans and nuts, to ease your pain

7. Rubbing clove oil relieves arthritis pain.

8. Soaking and eating one teaspoon of fenugreek or fenugreek powder daily cures arthritis.

9. Roast fenugreek in some ghee and then add jaggery and ghee to it and make ladoo. Eating this ladoo for eight to ten days

cures back pain and arthritis, relaxes stiff limbs and relieves tingling in hands and feet.

10.   Exercises for back pain:

(a)   Back extension (Bhujangasana): 10 times with 2-3 seconds of hold in each repetition.

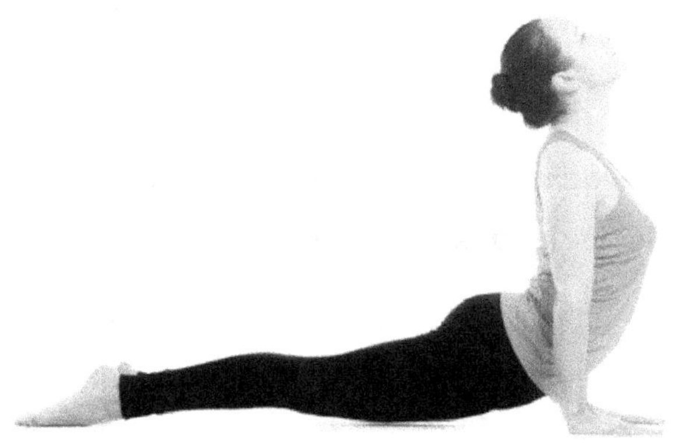

(b) Child pose: 5 to 10 times with 5 seconds hold in each repetition

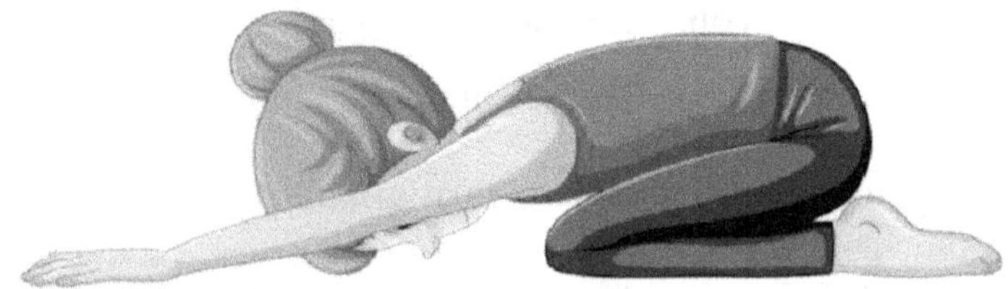

11.   Massage from 'point 2 to 1 to 2' to relieve back pain

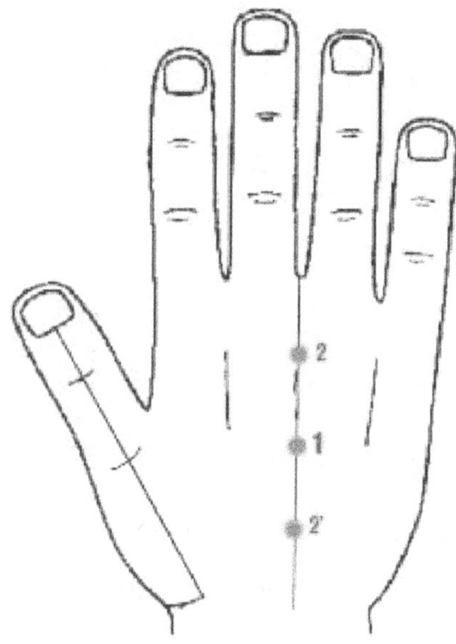

12.   DONT's for Back pain:

- Don't perform a full sit-up. The back is under too much stress from this.

- Avoid performing stretches that require you to extend your legs straight to touch your toes. Your already aching back muscles may suffer from this.

- Avoid Jogging: Jogging is a fantastic aerobic activity, but high impact exercises can be painful for your back.

- DON'T go too far. Know what hurts and what doesn't, and stay away from exercises that aggravate your pain.

Chapter 6: Instant Remedies for Migraine

Lifestyle choices that promote overall good health also can reduce the number of migraines you have and lessen the migraine pain.

Home remedies to treat migraine:

1. A dark, quite room - Calm environment and turning off lights helps since Light and sound can make migraine pain worse. Relax in a dark, quiet room. Sleep if you can.

2. Temperature therapy - Apply hot or cold compresses to your head or neck. Ice packs helps to reduce the pain. Hot packs helps to relax tense muscles.

3. Improve sleep habits - Establish regular sleeping hours . Naps longer than 20 to 30 minutes may interfere with nighttime sleep.

4. Reduce distraction: Don't watch television or take work materials to bed.

5. Exercise regularly

6. While exercising, your body releases certain chemicals that block pain signals to your brain. These chemicals also help

reduce anxiety and depression — two conditions that can make migraines worse.

7. Stress management: stress often goes hand in hand with migraine - (1) Simplify your life (2) Manage your time wisely (3) Take a break: You can do slow stretches or a quick walk (4) Stay positive (5) Relax: Deep breathing from your diaphragm can help you relax. Focus on inhaling and exhaling slowly and deeply for at least 10 minutes every day.

8. Keep a migraine diary: You should know what triggers your migraines. note when your migraines started, what you were doing at the time, how long they lasted and what, if anything, provided relief.

9.

Acupressure Points For Migraine Headache

ALL STRESS GATHERS AT THESE SPOTS

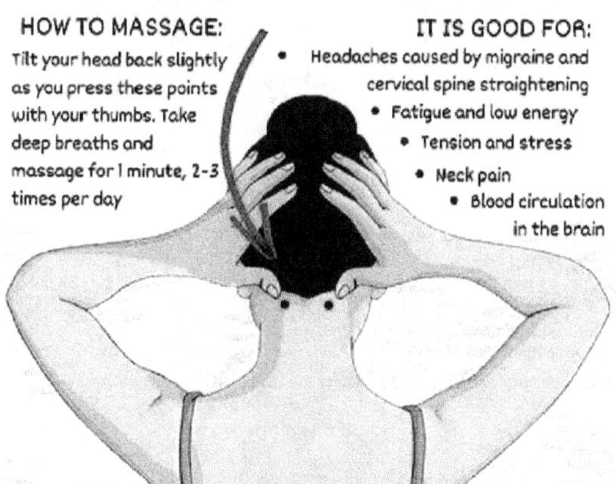

10.

HOW TO DO
MAHASIRS MUDRA
FOR HEADACHE

11.

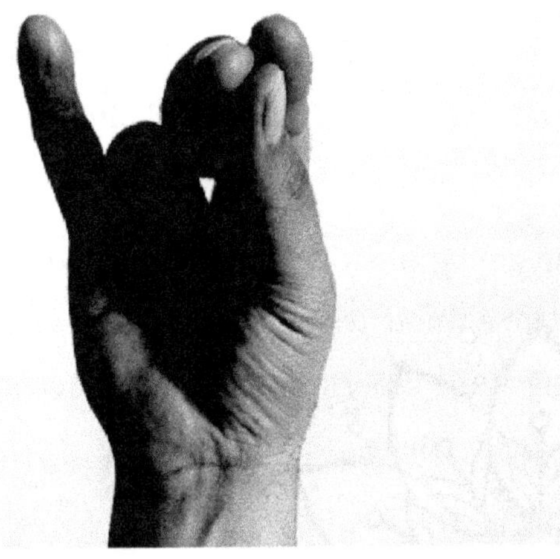

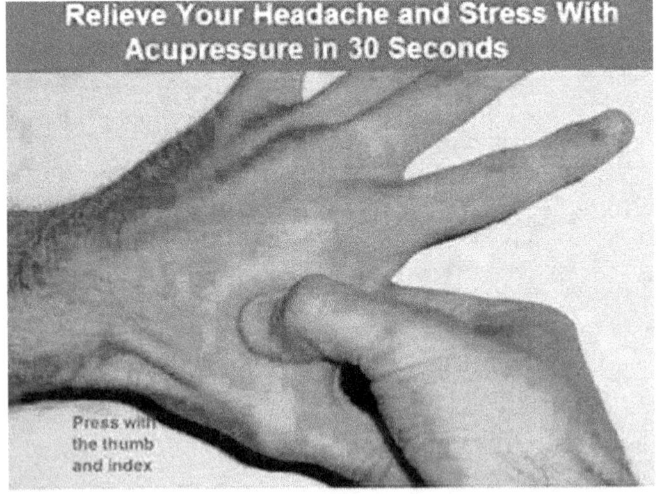
Relieve Your Headache and Stress With
Acupressure in 30 Seconds
Press with
the thumb
and index

12.   Nabhi kriya: Lavender oil may help relieve stress, anxiety, and headaches

13.   Massage: Massaging the muscles in the neck and shoulders helps to relieve tension and reduce migraine pain. Massage may also reduce stress.

14.   Yoga for migraine:

a. Child pose

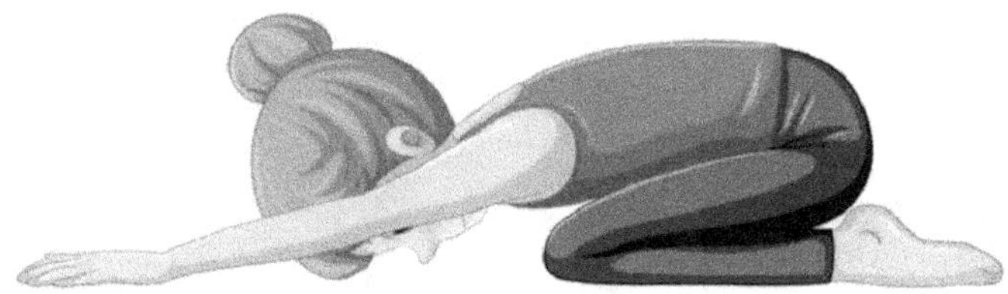

b. Downward facing dog

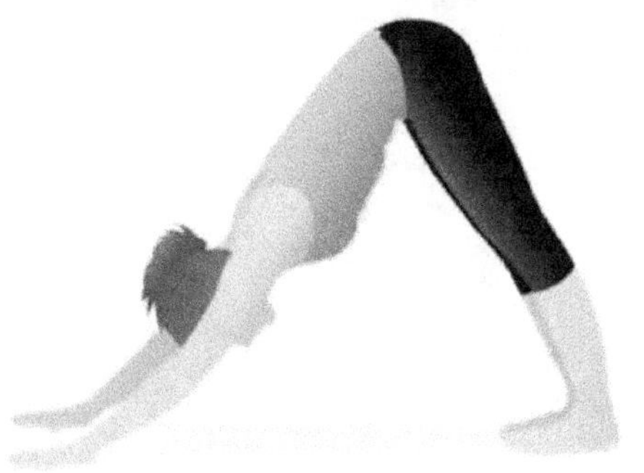

c. Corpse pose

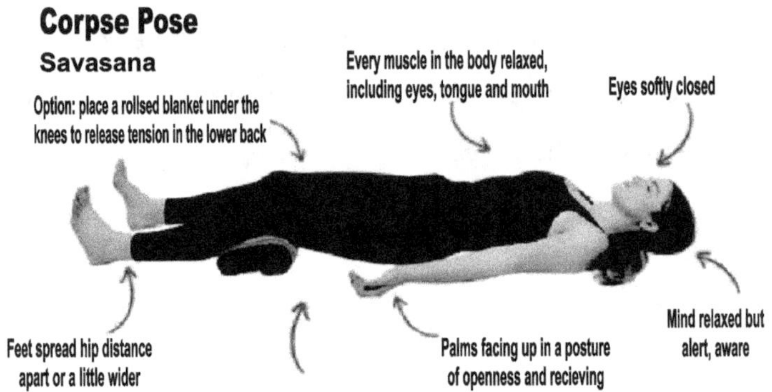

d. Vajrasana

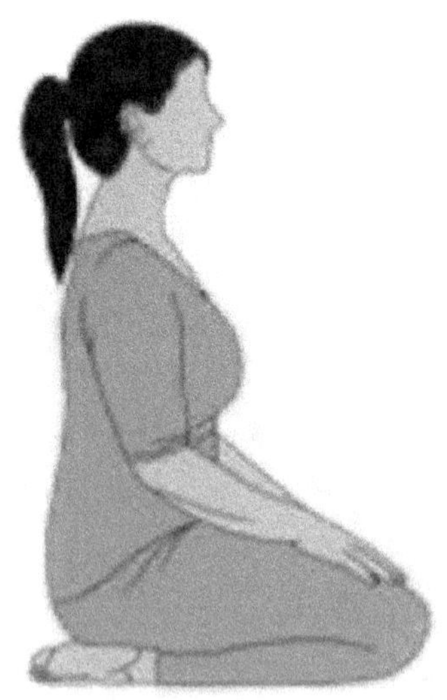

e. Pranayama

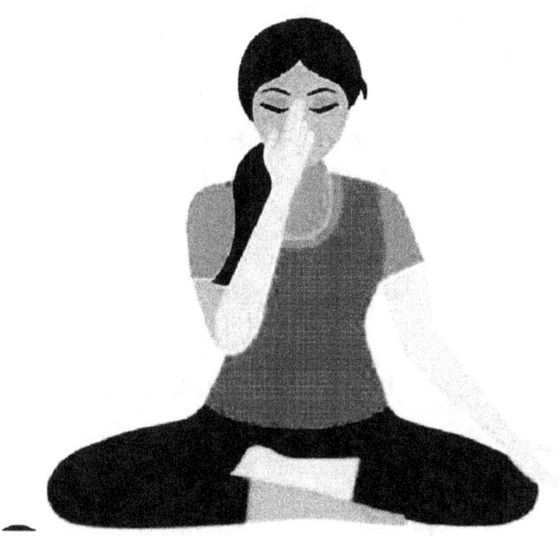

15.   Foods to avoid: Alcohol, especially red wine. Caffeine, which is in coffee, tea, colas, and other sodas. Foods made with nitrates, such as pepperoni, hot dogs, and lunch meats. Dried fruits.

16.   Figs in particular are a great fruit to choose, due to their high potassium content, to help keep migraines at bay. Potassium is an electrolyte that helps boost hydration levels and can reduce muscle cramping and fatigue. Bananas are another potassium-rich fruit.

17.   Magnesium, omega-3 fatty acids, keto-friendly foods, and caffeine may all help prevent migraine attacks. Consider adding foods like dark leafy greens, avocado, and fish to your diet.

Chapter 7: Instant Remedies for Urine Problems

1. Taking amla powder with ghee and jaggery daily cures all urinary problems.

2. If the urine flow is not proper then having mix honey in cardamom powder will make the urine clear and free.

3. By adding one gram of baking soda in 100 ml of milk and drinking it twice a day, urine will be free and urinary inflammation will be removed. Drinking boiled barley water clears urine and cures urinary inflammation.

4. Drinking sugarcane juice relieves urination, relieves inflammation and if there is blood in the urine, it also gets cured.

5. Taking cardamom powder with amla powder or in amla juice relieves urinary irritation. If you have to urinate frequently, take carrom seeds and sesame seeds in equal proportions and chew a lot in the morning and evening.

6. Taking sugar in ginger juice and drinking it in the morning and at night gives relief if you have to urinate frequently.

7.   Mixing mixture of half a teaspoon of carrom seeds and half a teaspoon of jaggery in the morning and evening relieves frequent urination.

8.   Foods that can help in urine problems : Pears, Bananas, Green beans, Winter squash, Potatoes, Lean proteins, Whole grains

9.   Follow a healthy eating plan

   • Drink enough liquids

   • Change your bathroom habits

   • Quit smoking

   • Avoid constipation

   • Do pelvic floor muscle exercises

10.   Kegel exercises can prevent or control urinary incontinence and other pelvic floor problems.

11.

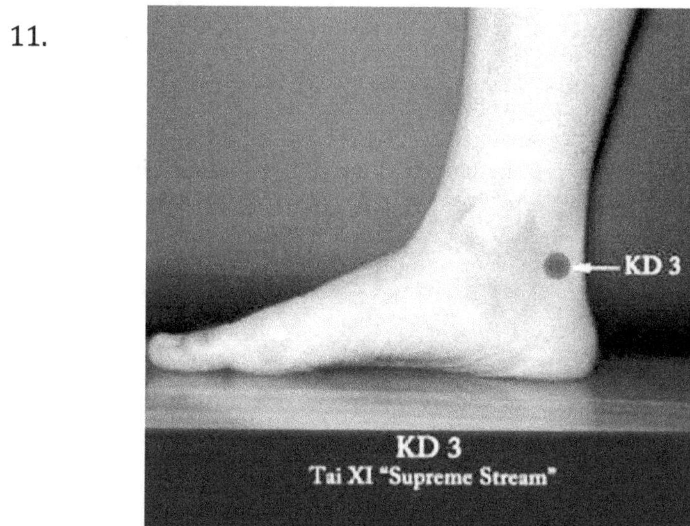

Gently press this point 5 to 7 times for 1 minute for any urinary problems

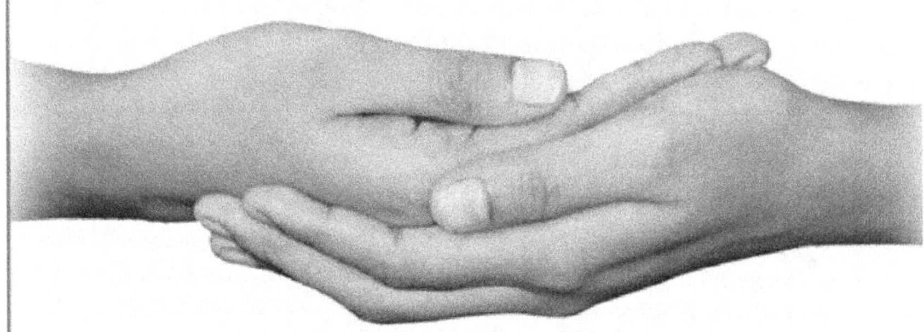

www.ingramcontent.com/pod-product-compliance
Lightning Source LLC
Chambersburg PA
CBHW050817160726
48004CB00002B/886